PANCREATIC CANCER HANDBOOK

A Comprehensive Guide for the Newly Diagnosed Patients and Caregivers

Dr. Mira Langford

Disclaimer

The information provided here is based on thorough research but not intended as a substitute for professional diagnosis, treatment, or care. Consult your physician or qualified healthcare provider for any medical concerns. Please note, this resource is not a remedy but intended for management purposes only. Individual responses to treatment may vary, and personalized medical guidance is essential for proper diagnosis, treatment, and management of health conditions.

Table of Contents

Introduction

Pancreatic cancer is a complex and challenging disease that requires a clear understanding of its nature, treatment options, and management strategies. This guide serves as a comprehensive resource, offering detailed information to help readers navigate the many aspects of pancreatic cancer.

From the basics of diagnosis and staging to the latest advancements in treatment, this book provides evidence-based insights for anyone seeking to deepen their understanding of the condition. It also addresses critical areas such as nutrition, symptom management, and emotional well-being, ensuring a holistic approach to care.

Whether used as a reference or read cover to cover, this guide is designed to educate, inform, and empower individuals as they explore the path forward.

Why This Book?

A diagnosis of pancreatic cancer is life-changing and often overwhelming. For many, it brings a whirlwind of emotions—fear, confusion, and uncertainty about what lies ahead. This book was created to provide clarity, guidance, and support for newly diagnosed patients and their families.

Pancreatic cancer can be challenging to understand and treat, but knowledge is a powerful tool. The more you know about your condition, treatment options, and supportive resources, the better equipped you will be to make informed decisions. This guide is designed to serve as a trusted companion, offering both medical information and practical strategies to help you navigate this journey with confidence.

A Message of Hope and Guidance for the Newly Diagnosed

While a diagnosis of pancreatic cancer can feel daunting, it is important to know that progress is being made every day in the understanding and treatment of this disease. Advances in surgery, chemotherapy, and personalized medicine are providing new avenues for treatment and improving outcomes for many patients.

This book aims to be more than just a source of information—it is a beacon of hope. You are not alone in this fight. By taking proactive steps, seeking the right care, and leaning on the support of loved ones and healthcare professionals, you can face this challenge with strength and determination.

Understanding Your Diagnosis: A First Step to Empowerment Hearing the words "you have pancreatic cancer" is one of life's most difficult moments. It's natural to feel uncertain or even powerless in the face of such news. However, understanding your diagnosis is the first step in reclaiming control.

This guide will help you comprehend:

- *What pancreatic cancer is*: Understanding the biology and behavior of the disease.
- *What stage you are in:* Knowing whether the cancer is localized, has spread regionally, or has metastasized.
- *Your treatment options:* Learning about surgery, chemotherapy, radiation, and new therapies.
- *What to expect moving forward:* Preparing for the journey ahead, from initial consultations to treatment and beyond.

Empowerment comes from knowledge, and by understanding your condition, you can actively participate in your care plan and advocate for the best possible outcomes.

How to Use This Book

This book is structured to serve as a practical and comprehensive guide, with each chapter addressing a critical aspect of pancreatic cancer care. Here's how to get the most from it:

- *Start with the basics:* If you're newly diagnosed, begin with the first chapters to understand what pancreatic cancer is, how it's diagnosed, and what the staging means for you.

- *Explore treatment options:* Read the sections on surgical and non-surgical treatments to learn what approaches may be available to you.
- *Focus on holistic care:* The chapters on nutrition, emotional well-being, and palliative care provide practical tips for improving your quality of life.
- *Use it as a reference:* If specific questions arise during your journey, revisit relevant sections for guidance.
- *Leverage the appendices:* Explore the glossary, FAQs, and resource list for additional support.

This book is designed to be your guide at every step, whether you're seeking answers to pressing questions, preparing for a medical appointment, or looking for ways to improve your well-being. Keep it close as a source of reliable information and encouragement.

Part 1: The Basics of Pancreatic Cancer

Chapter 1: What is Pancreatic Cancer?

Understanding the Pancreas and Its Role in the Body

The pancreas is a vital organ located behind the stomach, playing a crucial role in both digestion and regulation of blood sugar. It is involved in two primary functions:

- ***Exocrine Function:*** The majority of the pancreas is made up of exocrine cells that produce digestive enzymes. These enzymes are released into the small intestine, where they help break down food, enabling the body to absorb nutrients.

- ***Endocrine Function:*** The pancreas also contains clusters of cells called islets of Langerhans, which produce hormones like insulin and glucagon. These hormones are essential for regulating blood sugar levels and maintaining energy balance in the body.

Pancreatic cancer arises when cells in the pancreas begin to grow uncontrollably, forming a tumor that disrupts these essential functions. Understanding the pancreas' role helps to recognize the complex ways pancreatic cancer can affect overall health.

Types of Pancreatic Cancer

Pancreatic cancer is primarily classified based on the type of cells from which it originates. There are two main types:

Exocrine Pancreatic Cancer (Adenocarcinoma):
The most common form of pancreatic cancer, accounting for approximately 90% of cases, is pancreatic ductal adenocarcinoma (PDAC). This cancer arises from the exocrine cells that line the ducts of the pancreas, which transport digestive enzymes. It is often diagnosed at an advanced stage because it grows silently and shows few symptoms in its early stages.

Endocrine Pancreatic Cancer (Pancreatic Neuroendocrine Tumors):
These tumors arise from the endocrine cells, which produce hormones. Although much less common, pancreatic neuroendocrine tumors (PNETs) tend to grow more slowly than adenocarcinomas and may sometimes be functional, meaning they can produce excess hormones that lead to symptoms related to hormone imbalances (e.g., insulin, glucagon). PNETs are often more treatable and may have a better prognosis than exocrine tumors, depending on their size and spread.

Exocrine Tumors vs. Endocrine Tumors

The distinction between exocrine and endocrine pancreatic cancers is crucial for understanding the disease's pathology and treatment approaches.

- ***Exocrine Tumors (Pancreatic Ductal Adenocarcinoma):*** These tumors originate from the ducts of the pancreas and are most commonly diagnosed in the later stages due to the pancreas' deep location in the abdomen. As a result, the disease tends to be more aggressive and is less likely to be cured through surgery once it has spread.

- ***Endocrine Tumors (Pancreatic Neuroendocrine Tumors):*** These tumors are rarer and form from the hormone-producing cells of the pancreas. Depending on whether the tumors are functional (producing hormones) or non-functional, the clinical course can vary. Non-functional tumors are typically diagnosed at a later stage, but functional tumors often present earlier due to the symptoms caused by hormone imbalances. Treatment for these tumors can be more diverse, ranging from surgery to targeted therapies.

Causes and Risk Factors

The exact cause of pancreatic cancer remains largely unknown, but there are several factors that increase the likelihood of developing the disease. These factors are categorized into genetic predisposition and lifestyle/environmental triggers.

Genetic Predisposition

1. Inherited Genetic Mutations:

Certain genetic mutations increase the risk of pancreatic cancer. These can be inherited in families, especially when multiple relatives are diagnosed with pancreatic cancer or other related cancers (e.g., breast, ovarian, or colorectal cancer). Some of the more common genetic syndromes associated with pancreatic cancer include:

- **Hereditary Pancreatitis:** Chronic inflammation of the pancreas increases the risk of pancreatic cancer.
- **BRCA1 and BRCA2 mutations:** These mutations, often associated with breast and ovarian cancers, can also increase the risk of pancreatic cancer.
- **Lynch Syndrome**: Also known as hereditary nonpolyposis colorectal cancer (HNPCC), this genetic condition increases the risk of several cancers, including pancreatic cancer.
- **Familial Atypical Multiple Mole Melanoma Syndrome (FAMMM):** Involves mutations that increase the risk of melanoma and pancreatic cancer.

2. Genetic Alterations in the Tumor:

Even in the absence of inherited mutations, cancers of the pancreas often exhibit mutations in specific genes, such as KRAS, TP53, and SMAD4, which can drive the progression of the disease. Advances in genetic research are helping to better understand how these mutations contribute to cancer development and provide potential targets for therapy.

Lifestyle and Environmental Triggers

Several lifestyle and environmental factors have been identified as increasing the risk of pancreatic cancer:

Tobacco Use:
- Smoking is one of the most significant risk factors for pancreatic cancer, responsible for approximately 20-30% of cases. The harmful chemicals in tobacco smoke can damage pancreatic cells, leading to cancer development.

Diet and Obesity:
- A diet high in red and processed meats, along with a low intake of fruits and vegetables, has been associated with an increased risk of pancreatic cancer. Obesity, particularly abdominal obesity, is another significant risk factor, as excess body fat can lead to increased insulin levels, which may promote tumor growth.

Chronic Pancreatitis:

- Long-term inflammation of the pancreas (chronic pancreatitis) significantly increases the risk of pancreatic cancer. Chronic pancreatitis can result from genetic conditions, heavy alcohol consumption, or other factors.

Diabetes:

- People with diabetes, especially those diagnosed with diabetes later in life, have a higher risk of developing pancreatic cancer. The relationship between diabetes and pancreatic cancer is complex; in some cases, pancreatic cancer may lead to the development of diabetes due to the tumor's effect on insulin production.

Alcohol Consumption:

- Heavy and prolonged alcohol consumption is linked to an increased risk of pancreatic cancer, particularly in individuals with a history of chronic pancreatitis.

Exposure to Certain Chemicals:

- Occupational exposure to certain chemicals, such as those used in the petroleum, chemical, and leather industries, may increase the risk of pancreatic cancer. Long-term exposure to carcinogens, particularly in industrial settings, is an established environmental risk factor.

Pancreatic cancer is a multifactorial disease with both genetic and environmental risk factors contributing to its development. Understanding the pancreas' role in the body, distinguishing between the different types of pancreatic cancer, and identifying the risk factors are essential for early detection and intervention. While some risk factors are non-modifiable, such as genetic predispositions, lifestyle changes, such as smoking cessation, a healthy diet, and maintaining a healthy weight, can help reduce the risk of developing pancreatic cancer. Advances in research continue to improve our understanding of the disease and offer hope for better treatments and outcomes.

Chapter 2: Recognizing Symptoms and Seeking Help

Early Warning Signs

Pancreatic cancer is notoriously difficult to detect in its early stages because it often does not cause noticeable symptoms until it has advanced. However, there are some early warning signs that may indicate the presence of the disease. It is important to note that these symptoms can also be caused by other, less serious conditions. Nonetheless, if these signs persist or worsen, seeking medical attention is crucial.

Unexplained Weight Loss:
- Sudden and unexplained weight loss is one of the most common early signs of pancreatic cancer. This may occur due to a combination of factors, including the body's inability to absorb nutrients effectively and changes in metabolism caused by the cancer.

Loss of Appetite:
- A diminished appetite or feeling full quickly after eating even small amounts of food is often associated with pancreatic cancer. This symptom may arise due to changes in the pancreas's ability to produce

digestive enzymes, leading to poor digestion and early satiety.

Digestive Issues:
- Difficulty in digesting food, particularly fatty foods, may occur early in pancreatic cancer. This is often due to the pancreas' reduced ability to secrete digestive enzymes, which are necessary for breaking down fats and other nutrients. This can lead to bloating, gas, and indigestion.

Jaundice (Yellowing of the Skin and Eyes):
- Jaundice occurs when the tumor obstructs the bile duct, leading to a buildup of bilirubin in the blood. This results in yellowing of the skin and the whites of the eyes. Jaundice is often accompanied by dark urine and pale-colored stools and can be one of the first signs that prompts individuals to seek medical care.

Pain in the Upper Abdomen or Back:
- Pain in the upper abdomen, which may radiate to the back, can be an early symptom of pancreatic cancer. This pain may be dull or constant, and in some cases, it can be relieved by leaning forward or sitting up. The pain may worsen after eating or lying down.

New Onset Diabetes or Worsening of Existing Diabetes:
- Pancreatic cancer can affect insulin production, leading to new-onset diabetes or the worsening of existing diabetes. Elevated blood sugar levels that are

difficult to control, despite treatment, can be an
indicator of underlying pancreatic disease.

Fatty Stool (Steatorrhea):

- Fatty stools, which are pale, foul-smelling, and
  difficult to flush, can occur if the pancreas is not
  producing enough digestive enzymes. These stools
  may float and leave an oily residue in the toilet bowl,
  which can be an early sign of pancreatic insufficiency
  related to cancer.

Symptoms of Advanced Pancreatic Cancer

As pancreatic cancer progresses, it becomes more
symptomatic and can lead to additional complications. These
symptoms are often more pronounced and affect various
aspects of the body's function. In advanced stages, the cancer
may have spread to other organs, such as the liver, lungs, or
peritoneum, and additional signs may include:

Worsening Abdominal or Back Pain:

- In more advanced stages, the pain associated with
  pancreatic cancer may become more severe and
  persistent. It may also spread to the back or other
  areas of the body as the tumor grows or spreads to
  nearby structures.

Severe Weight Loss and Malnutrition:

- As the cancer progresses, patients may experience
  even more significant weight loss and muscle
  wasting. This is due to the cancer's impact on the

digestive system, as well as the body's increased metabolic demand in the presence of the tumor.

Ascites (Abdominal Fluid Build-up):

- As the cancer spreads to the peritoneum or liver, fluid may begin to accumulate in the abdomen, causing swelling, discomfort, and difficulty breathing. This is known as ascites and is a sign of advanced disease.

Obstructive Jaundice:

- In the later stages of pancreatic cancer, jaundice may become more pronounced due to the tumor's obstruction of the bile duct. The skin and eyes may become visibly yellow, and additional complications, such as itching and liver dysfunction, may arise.

Bowel Obstruction:

- A tumor that grows in or near the intestines can cause partial or complete bowel obstruction. Symptoms may include severe nausea, vomiting, inability to pass gas or stool, and bloating. This can be a serious complication that requires immediate medical intervention.

Fatigue and General Malaise:

- As pancreatic cancer advances, individuals often experience profound fatigue and a general sense of unwellness. This is due to the body's ongoing struggle with the cancer, including the effects of metabolic changes, nutrient deficiencies, and the stress on various organ systems.

Liver Dysfunction:

- If the cancer spreads to the liver, it may cause liver dysfunction, resulting in elevated liver enzymes, jaundice, and changes in clotting factors. These can lead to bleeding issues or other severe complications that require urgent medical attention.

Mental Confusion or Disorientation:

- As the disease progresses, some individuals may experience confusion or changes in mental status due to liver dysfunction, electrolyte imbalances, or the spread of cancer to the brain or other parts of the nervous system.

The Importance of Timely Diagnosis

Timely diagnosis is crucial in the management of pancreatic cancer, as it is one of the deadliest cancers with a generally poor prognosis. Early detection can significantly improve treatment outcomes, allowing for the possibility of surgical intervention, more effective chemotherapy, and potentially better long-term survival. Unfortunately, because the symptoms often do not appear until the disease is advanced, many cases are not diagnosed until the cancer has spread beyond the pancreas.

The key to improving outcomes lies in recognizing early warning signs and seeking medical attention promptly. Even though early-stage pancreatic cancer can be asymptomatic or present with vague symptoms, individuals who experience persistent digestive issues, unexplained weight loss, jaundice, or new-onset diabetes should consult with a healthcare provider. In some cases, routine imaging tests or screenings for high-risk populations (such as individuals with a family history of pancreatic cancer) can lead to earlier detection.

Diagnostic methods, including blood tests (such as CA 19-9), imaging techniques (CT scans, MRIs), and biopsies, play a critical role in confirming the presence of pancreatic cancer and determining its stage. The earlier the cancer is detected, the more options there are for treatment, which may include surgery, chemotherapy, and radiation therapy, aimed at controlling or removing the tumor.

Ultimately, early diagnosis increases the chances for better outcomes and offers patients the opportunity to explore a wider range of treatment options, which may improve quality of life and extend survival. Recognizing symptoms early and seeking help from a medical professional can make a significant difference in the trajectory of the disease.

Chapter 3: Diagnosis and Staging Explained

Diagnostic Tests and What They Reveal

Diagnosing pancreatic cancer involves a combination of clinical evaluation, laboratory tests, and imaging techniques. These tests help to confirm the presence of cancer, determine its location, and assess how far it has spread. Early and accurate diagnosis is crucial for developing an effective treatment plan.

1. Blood Tests:

Blood tests play an important role in diagnosing pancreatic cancer, though they cannot confirm the disease on their own. They help identify potential biomarkers that indicate the presence of cancer, monitor organ function, and rule out other conditions.

CA 19-9:

- One of the most commonly used blood tests for pancreatic cancer is the measurement of CA 19-9, a tumor marker that is often elevated in patients with pancreatic cancer. However, CA 19-9 levels can also be elevated in other conditions, such as benign pancreatic disorders or liver disease, so it is not diagnostic on its own. A normal CA 19-9 level does not rule out cancer, and elevated levels may not necessarily indicate pancreatic cancer.

Liver Function Tests:
- Since pancreatic cancer can spread to the liver, liver function tests may show abnormalities in enzymes such as ALT, AST, and alkaline phosphatase. These tests can help assess whether the liver has been affected by the tumor or its spread.

Glucose and Other Metabolic Tests:
- Pancreatic cancer can impact insulin production, leading to abnormal blood glucose levels. Elevated glucose levels may suggest an issue with pancreatic function, including the possibility of a tumor.

2. Imaging Tests:
Imaging plays a crucial role in identifying the tumor, its size, location, and whether it has spread to other parts of the body. The most commonly used imaging techniques for pancreatic cancer include:

Computed Tomography (CT) Scan:
- CT scans are often the first imaging test performed to evaluate pancreatic cancer. A CT scan provides detailed images of the abdomen and allows doctors to visualize the tumor, assess whether it has invaded nearby organs, and check for any signs of metastasis to distant organs like the liver or lungs.

Magnetic Resonance Imaging (MRI):

- An MRI uses magnetic fields to produce high-resolution images of the pancreas and surrounding tissues. It is particularly useful in identifying small tumors and in assessing the extent of cancer spread, especially to the bile ducts or liver.

Endoscopic Ultrasound (EUS):

- EUS involves passing a thin, flexible tube with an ultrasound device through the stomach to obtain detailed images of the pancreas. This test allows for a closer look at the tumor and can also help guide a biopsy if needed. EUS is particularly helpful for detecting small tumors that may not be visible on other imaging modalities.

Positron Emission Tomography (PET) Scan:

- PET scans are sometimes used to assess whether pancreatic cancer has spread to other parts of the body. A PET scan detects areas of high metabolic activity, which is characteristic of cancer cells. It is often used in combination with CT or MRI to provide a more comprehensive view of the disease.

3. Biopsy:

A biopsy is the definitive test for confirming the diagnosis of pancreatic cancer. It involves the removal of a small sample of tissue from the tumor for examination under a microscope. The biopsy can be performed using several methods, including:

Endoscopic Ultrasound-Guided Biopsy:

- This is a common technique where an ultrasound probe is inserted through the stomach to obtain a tissue sample from the pancreas.

CT-guided Biopsy:

- If the tumor is accessible, a needle may be inserted into the tumor through the skin to collect tissue for biopsy, guided by a CT scan.

Laparoscopy:

- In some cases, a minimally invasive surgical procedure called laparoscopy may be used to obtain tissue samples. This involves inserting a small camera and surgical tools through small incisions in the abdomen to directly visualize and biopsy the tumor.

While a biopsy is the most accurate method for diagnosing pancreatic cancer, it is not always feasible, particularly if the tumor is in a difficult location. In such cases, a combination of imaging and blood tests may be used to establish the diagnosis.

Understanding Stages and How They Guide Treatment

The stage of pancreatic cancer refers to how far the cancer has spread from its original location. Staging is crucial for determining the most appropriate treatment approach, as it helps guide decisions about surgery, chemotherapy, radiation, and other therapies.

Pancreatic cancer is typically staged using the TNM system, which assesses:

- *T (Tumor):* The size of the primary tumor and whether it has invaded nearby tissues.
- *N (Nodes):* Whether cancer has spread to nearby lymph nodes.
- *M (Metastasis)*: Whether cancer has spread to distant organs.

The stages of pancreatic cancer range from *stage I (localized) to stage IV (advanced metastatic disease)*, with subcategories in between. Here's a breakdown of the stages:

Stage I:
- At this stage, the cancer is confined to the pancreas and has not spread to nearby tissues or lymph nodes. Treatment may involve surgery to remove the tumor, potentially followed by chemotherapy or radiation.

Stage II:
- In stage II, the cancer may have spread to nearby tissues or lymph nodes but is still considered localized. Surgery is often the primary treatment option, although chemotherapy and radiation may be recommended before or after surgery to improve outcomes.

Stage III:

- Stage III pancreatic cancer indicates that the tumor has spread to nearby blood vessels or other structures, making it difficult or impossible to surgically remove the tumor. Treatment options at this stage typically involve chemotherapy, possibly combined with radiation therapy, to shrink the tumor and manage symptoms.

Stage IV:

- Stage IV is the most advanced stage, indicating that cancer has spread (metastasized) to distant organs such as the liver, lungs, or peritoneum. At this stage, pancreatic cancer is generally considered incurable, and treatment is focused on palliative care, symptom management, and improving quality of life. Chemotherapy and targeted therapies may be used to control the growth of the tumor and extend survival.

Staging helps oncologists recommend the most effective treatment strategy and gives patients a clearer understanding of the disease's prognosis. However, each case is unique, and treatment plans are often personalized based on individual factors such as age, overall health, and specific tumor characteristics.

Genetic Testing: Its Role in Treatment Choices

Genetic testing plays an increasingly important role in the diagnosis and treatment of pancreatic cancer. It involves analyzing the genetic makeup of both the patient's cancer and, in some cases, the patient's normal tissue to identify mutations or alterations that may influence treatment decisions.

Identification of Targeted Therapy Options:
- Advances in precision medicine have led to the development of targeted therapies that specifically address genetic mutations driving the growth of certain cancers. For example, tumors with mutations in the BRCA1 or BRCA2 genes, which are commonly associated with hereditary breast and ovarian cancers, may respond to therapies like PARP inhibitors. Other genetic mutations, such as those in the KRAS gene, may affect treatment options and provide insight into the aggressiveness of the disease.

Personalized Treatment Plans:
- By identifying specific mutations, oncologists can design treatment regimens tailored to the individual's genetic profile, potentially improving the effectiveness of therapy. For example, patients with specific mutations may be eligible for clinical trials of new targeted therapies or immunotherapies that are not available to all patients.

Testing for Genetic Syndromes:
- For individuals with a family history of pancreatic cancer or related cancers, genetic testing can also identify inherited syndromes such as Lynch syndrome, Peutz-Jeghers syndrome, or hereditary pancreatitis. Identifying these syndromes can help guide treatment choices and inform family members about their own cancer risk.

Comprehensive Genomic Profiling:
- Comprehensive genomic profiling tests analyze the entire genetic makeup of a patient's tumor, providing a detailed view of the mutations and alterations present. This information can help determine which therapies may be most effective and guide participation in clinical trials.

Genetic testing is not routinely performed on all pancreatic cancer patients, but it is becoming an increasingly important tool in the management of the disease. It allows for a more personalized approach to treatment, which may improve outcomes and help identify patients who might benefit from specific therapies.

Part 2: Treatment Options and Medical Management

Chapter 4: Surgical Options

When Surgery is Possible

Surgery is the primary treatment option for pancreatic cancer when the tumor is localized and can be completely removed. However, not all patients are candidates for surgery, and the decision to undergo surgery depends on several factors, including the stage of cancer, tumor location, involvement of surrounding blood vessels, and the overall health of the patient. The primary goal of surgery is to remove the tumor and, in some cases, surrounding tissues to achieve the best possible outcome.

In general, surgery is considered when the tumor is confined to the pancreas or has not spread to distant organs. The decision to proceed with surgery is typically made after careful evaluation using imaging techniques, biopsy results, and staging assessments. If the tumor has spread beyond the pancreas to vital structures such as major blood vessels or other organs, surgical options may be limited.

For patients who are candidates for surgery, a multidisciplinary team of oncologists, surgeons, and other healthcare professionals will assess the best surgical approach based on the individual case. Surgery may be followed by chemotherapy or radiation therapy to help eliminate any remaining cancer cells and reduce the risk of recurrence.

Types of Surgical Procedures

There are several types of surgical procedures used to treat pancreatic cancer, and the choice of surgery depends on the tumor's location, its extent, and other factors specific to the patient. The most common surgical procedures for pancreatic cancer include the Whipple procedure, distal pancreatectomy, and total pancreatectomy.

1. Whipple Procedure (Pancreaticoduodenectomy):

The Whipple procedure is the most common surgery performed for pancreatic cancer located in the head of the pancreas, which is the part closest to the duodenum (the first section of the small intestine). This complex surgery involves the removal of:

- The head of the pancreas
- The duodenum
- The gallbladder
- A portion of the bile duct
- The lymph nodes near the pancreas

In some cases, part of the stomach may also be removed. After the tumor is removed, the remaining parts of the pancreas, bile duct, and intestines are reconnected to allow for normal digestion.

The Whipple procedure is a highly intricate operation that requires specialized surgical expertise, as it involves removing and reconnecting critical structures in the abdomen. This surgery can provide the best chance for cure in patients with early-stage pancreatic cancer that has not spread to surrounding organs or blood vessels.

The Whipple procedure is associated with a relatively long recovery period and potential complications, but it remains the most effective option for patients with resectable tumors.

2. Distal Pancreatectomy:

Distal pancreatectomy is the surgical removal of the body and tail of the pancreas, typically performed when the tumor is located in these regions. This surgery is often used for pancreatic tumors that arise in the tail of the pancreas or when the cancer is localized to the body and tail of the organ.

In some cases, the spleen is also removed during this procedure if the tumor is close to the spleen. If the spleen is removed, the patient may be at a higher risk of infections and may need vaccinations or other treatments to help prevent infections in the future.

Distal pancreatectomy is generally considered for tumors that are confined to the body and tail of the pancreas and do not involve major blood vessels or nearby organs. It is less complex than the Whipple procedure but still requires careful planning to minimize complications and ensure complete tumor removal.

3. Total Pancreatectomy:

Total pancreatectomy involves the removal of the entire pancreas, as well as parts of the stomach, small intestine, and bile ducts, depending on the tumor's location. This procedure may be considered in cases where the cancer is widespread throughout the pancreas or when there is a high risk of recurrence despite removal of the tumor.

After a total pancreatectomy, patients will no longer have a pancreas and will require lifelong insulin therapy to manage blood sugar levels. Additionally, they will need enzyme replacement therapy to help with digestion, as the pancreas produces digestive enzymes essential for breaking down food. This surgery is more radical than the Whipple or distal pancreatectomy and carries a higher risk of complications, but it may be the best option for certain patients.

Recovery: What to Expect

Recovery after pancreatic surgery can be a lengthy and challenging process, and it varies depending on the type of surgery performed, the patient's overall health, and any complications that arise during the procedure. Understanding what to expect during recovery can help patients prepare for the process.

Hospital Stay:

After pancreatic surgery, patients typically stay in the hospital for several days to weeks, depending on the type of surgery and how well they are recovering. During this time, patients will be closely monitored for complications, such as infection, bleeding, or problems with digestion. Pain management, nutritional support, and physical therapy may be provided to help with recovery.

Pain Management:
Pain is a common part of recovery from pancreatic surgery, and patients will be given medications to manage it. This may include oral pain relievers or intravenous pain medications in the hospital. Pain management will be adjusted based on the patient's needs and may taper as the recovery process progresses.

Nutritional Support:
After pancreatic surgery, especially if a significant portion of the pancreas is removed, patients may experience difficulty digesting food. In some cases, patients may initially be unable to eat solid foods and may require feeding through a tube (such as a nasogastric tube or gastrostomy tube) until they are able to tolerate food orally. A dietitian will typically help patients with meal planning to ensure they receive adequate nutrition.

Patients may need to take pancreatic enzyme replacements to help with digestion, especially after procedures like the Whipple procedure or total pancreatectomy These enzymes aid in the breakdown of food and prevent malabsorption, a common issue after pancreatic surgery.

Physical Activity and Rehabilitation:
After surgery, patients will be encouraged to begin light physical activities as soon as possible to promote circulation, prevent blood clots, and enhance overall recovery. Physical therapy may be recommended to help with mobility and strength, particularly after more extensive surgeries like the

Whipple or total pancreatectomy. It may take several weeks to months to regain normal levels of energy and strength.

Complications and Long-term Care:
As with any major surgery, there are risks of complications, including infection, bleeding, or issues with digestion. Patients should be aware of the signs of infection, such as fever or redness around the surgical site, and seek medical attention promptly if any unusual symptoms occur.

Long-term follow-up care is important to monitor for any recurrence of pancreatic cancer, manage diabetes if the pancreas was removed, and ensure proper digestion and nutrition. Regular imaging tests, blood work, and clinical assessments will be part of ongoing care.

Emotional and Psychological Support:
Recovering from pancreatic surgery can be emotionally and psychologically challenging. The stresses of recovery, combined with the uncertainty of cancer treatment, may require psychological or counseling support. Support groups or therapy may help patients cope with the emotional aspects of recovery.

The recovery process from pancreatic surgery is individual, and patients will be closely monitored to ensure the best possible outcomes. With proper care and support, many patients can return to a good quality of life after surgery, although they may need to adjust to life with a modified digestive system and, in some cases, diabetes.

Chapter 5: Non-Surgical Treatments

Non-surgical treatments play a vital role in the management of pancreatic cancer, especially for patients whose tumors are inoperable, have spread to distant organs, or when surgery is not a viable option. These treatments aim to control the growth of the tumor, alleviate symptoms, and improve overall survival. The primary non-surgical treatments for pancreatic cancer are chemotherapy, radiation therapy, and in some cases, combination treatments.

Chemotherapy

Chemotherapy is the use of drugs to kill cancer cells or slow their growth by interfering with their ability to divide and reproduce. It is one of the most commonly used treatments for pancreatic cancer, particularly for advanced stages or when the cancer cannot be surgically removed. Chemotherapy may be used as the primary treatment or in conjunction with surgery, radiation, or other therapies.

Common Drugs Used for Pancreatic Cancer
Several chemotherapy drugs are used to treat pancreatic cancer, either alone or in combination with other agents. The choice of chemotherapy regimen depends on the individual's specific diagnosis, cancer stage, and overall health.

Gemcitabine (Gemzar):

- Gemcitabine is one of the most commonly used chemotherapy drugs for pancreatic cancer. It is often used as the standard treatment for advanced pancreatic cancer and has been shown to improve survival rates, particularly when combined with other drugs or treatments. Gemcitabine works by interfering with DNA replication, preventing cancer cells from dividing and growing.

FOLFIRINOX:

- FOLFIRINOX is a combination chemotherapy regimen that includes fluorouracil (5-FU), oxaliplatin, irinotecan, and leucovorin. It is generally used for patients with a good performance status and is considered more effective than gemcitabine alone in treating pancreatic cancer. However, it can be associated with more severe side effects, so it is not appropriate for all patients.

Capecitabine (Xeloda):

- Capecitabine is an oral chemotherapy drug that is metabolized into 5-FU in the body. It may be used in combination with gemcitabine or other chemotherapy drugs to treat pancreatic cancer. It is often used when a patient cannot tolerate intravenous treatments or as part of a combination regimen.

Nab-paclitaxel (Abraxane):

- Nab-paclitaxel is a formulation of paclitaxel bound to albumin, which enhances its ability to penetrate tumors. When combined with gemcitabine, it has been shown to improve outcomes for patients with advanced pancreatic cancer. It works by interfering with cell division and stabilizing microtubules, preventing cancer cells from proliferating.

Other Chemotherapy Drugs:
- Other chemotherapy agents, such as 5-FU, mitomycin, and cisplatin, may also be used depending on the specific clinical scenario, although they are less commonly used in current standard regimens.

Managing Side Effects
Chemotherapy can cause side effects due to its impact on both cancerous and normal healthy cells. The severity and type of side effects vary depending on the drugs used, the dose, and the individual's overall health. Common side effects of chemotherapy for pancreatic cancer include:

- **Fatigue**: Fatigue is one of the most common side effects of chemotherapy. Patients may feel extremely tired, which can affect their ability to perform daily activities.
- **Nausea and Vomiting:** Many chemotherapy drugs cause nausea and vomiting, though this can usually be controlled with anti-nausea medications.
- **Hair Loss:** Some chemotherapy drugs, such as those in the FOLFIRINOX regimen, can lead to hair loss. This side effect is usually temporary.
- **Low Blood Counts:** Chemotherapy can lower the levels of red blood cells, white blood cells, and

platelets, leading to anemia, increased risk of infections, and bleeding. Regular blood tests are necessary to monitor these levels.

- **Diarrhea or Constipation:** Changes in bowel movements can occur due to the effect of chemotherapy on the digestive system.
- **Neuropathy:** Drugs like nab-paclitaxel and oxaliplatin can cause nerve damage, leading to symptoms like numbness, tingling, and weakness, particularly in the hands and feet.

Supportive medications, lifestyle adjustments, and close monitoring by the oncology team can help manage these side effects. In some cases, dose adjustments or changes in the treatment plan may be necessary.

Radiation Therapy

Radiation therapy uses high-energy rays, such as X-rays or protons, to kill or damage cancer cells. It is often used as a supplementary treatment alongside chemotherapy, especially for patients with localized pancreatic tumors. Radiation therapy can be used to shrink tumors before surgery, eliminate remaining cancer cells after surgery, or treat areas where cancer has spread, such as lymph nodes or nearby tissues.

How It Works and When It's Used

Radiation therapy works by damaging the DNA inside cancer cells, which prevents them from growing and dividing. Although radiation is effective at targeting cancer cells, it can also damage nearby healthy tissues, which is why its use is carefully planned and monitored.

Preoperative Radiation:

- Radiation therapy may be used before surgery to shrink the tumor, making it easier to remove. This is often done in combination with chemotherapy (chemoradiation) to increase effectiveness.

Postoperative Radiation:

- After surgery, radiation therapy may be used to eliminate any remaining cancer cells and reduce the risk of recurrence. This is typically part of a comprehensive treatment plan that also includes chemotherapy.

Palliative Radiation:

- For patients with advanced pancreatic cancer who are not candidates for surgery, radiation may be used to alleviate symptoms such as pain or blockages in the bile ducts or intestines. It can help relieve obstruction, improve jaundice, and reduce tumor size to provide symptomatic relief.

External Beam Radiation:

- The most common form of radiation therapy for pancreatic cancer is external beam radiation, where a machine directs focused radiation beams at the tumor from outside the body. Treatment is usually given in daily sessions over several weeks.

Stereotactic Body Radiation Therapy (SBRT):

- SBRT is a more advanced form of radiation that delivers a higher dose of radiation in fewer treatment sessions, often in five or fewer. It is particularly useful for patients with small, localized tumors that cannot be surgically removed.

Side Effects of Radiation Therapy

Radiation therapy is typically well-tolerated, but side effects can occur, particularly with extended courses of treatment. Common side effects include:

- **Fatigue:** Many patients experience tiredness or fatigue during radiation therapy.
- **Skin Irritation:** The area of the skin being treated may become red, irritated, or dry.
- **Digestive Issues:** Radiation targeting the pancreas may cause nausea, diarrhea, or changes in appetite, as the radiation can affect the surrounding gastrointestinal tract.
- **Pain or Discomfort:** Some patients may experience discomfort in the area being treated, particularly if the tumor is near sensitive structures.

Supportive care is available to manage side effects, and treatment plans are tailored to minimize exposure to healthy tissue.

Combination Treatments

In many cases, pancreatic cancer treatment involves a combination of chemotherapy, radiation therapy, and sometimes targeted therapies or immunotherapies. This approach can improve the overall effectiveness of treatment by attacking cancer cells through different mechanisms.

1. Chemoradiation (Chemotherapy + Radiation Therapy)
Chemoradiation, which combines chemotherapy with radiation therapy, is often used for patients with locally advanced pancreatic cancer or those who are not candidates for surgery. Chemotherapy drugs like gemcitabine or capecitabine can make cancer cells more sensitive to radiation, improving the likelihood of tumor shrinkage or control.

- *Neoadjuvant Chemoradiation*: This approach is used before surgery to shrink tumors, making them more resectable.
- *Adjuvant Chemoradiation*: This approach is used after surgery to eliminate remaining microscopic cancer cells and reduce the risk of recurrence.

2. Palliative Treatment
For patients with metastatic pancreatic cancer or those who are not candidates for surgery, combining chemotherapy with radiation therapy can help control tumor growth, alleviate symptoms, and extend life. These treatments may not cure the cancer but can improve quality of life by managing symptoms such as pain, bile duct obstruction, or intestinal blockages.

3. Targeted Therapies and Immunotherapies

In some cases, pancreatic cancer may be treated with targeted therapies or immunotherapies in combination with chemotherapy or radiation. These treatments target specific genetic mutations or proteins that drive cancer growth, offering a more personalized approach to treatment. Clinical trials exploring these combinations are ongoing, and some targeted agents may be approved for use in certain pancreatic cancer subtypes.

The goal of combination treatments is to maximize the efficacy of each treatment modality, often improving survival and reducing tumor burden. The exact combination used will depend on the patient's individual cancer characteristics, tumor stage, and overall health.

Non-surgical treatments for pancreatic cancer, including chemotherapy, radiation, and combination therapies, are essential components of the treatment landscape. The choice of treatment depends on the cancer's stage, the patient's response to prior therapies, and the overall treatment goals. By working with a multidisciplinary team, patients can receive the most appropriate and effective non-surgical treatment for their specific needs.

Chapter 6: Emerging Treatments and Advances in Care

The treatment landscape for pancreatic cancer has evolved significantly in recent years, with ongoing research into new therapies and improved methods of care. While traditional treatments such as surgery, chemotherapy, and radiation therapy remain the standard, emerging treatments like immunotherapy, targeted therapy, and advances in personalized medicine are offering new hope for patients. Clinical trials also continue to explore innovative approaches, potentially changing the way pancreatic cancer is treated in the future.

Immunotherapy and Targeted Therapy

Immunotherapy and targeted therapy represent two of the most promising areas of cancer research. Both aim to treat cancer more effectively and with fewer side effects compared to traditional treatments. These therapies focus on the unique biological aspects of cancer cells and the body's immune system to fight the disease.

1. Immunotherapy

Immunotherapy works by stimulating or enhancing the body's own immune system to recognize and attack cancer cells. The immune system normally identifies and destroys abnormal cells, but cancer cells often develop mechanisms to evade detection. Immunotherapy aims to overcome these defenses and enable the immune system to target and kill cancer cells more effectively.

Immune Checkpoint Inhibitors:

- Immune checkpoint inhibitors are a class of immunotherapy drugs that block specific proteins on cancer cells or immune cells, allowing the immune system to better recognize and attack tumors. Some of the most studied checkpoint inhibitors are those targeting PD-1 (programmed cell death protein 1) or PD-L1 (programmed death-ligand 1), which are proteins that help tumors evade immune surveillance. The most commonly used PD-1 inhibitors include pembrolizumab (Keytruda) and nivolumab (Opdivo). These inhibitors have shown promise in various cancers, though their success in pancreatic cancer has been limited so far, often requiring additional therapies to be fully effective.

Cancer Vaccines:

- Cancer vaccines aim to stimulate the immune system to target specific cancer cells. While not yet widely available, vaccines like GVAX are being studied in clinical trials for their potential to treat pancreatic cancer. These vaccines are designed to prompt the immune system to recognize tumor antigens, thus enhancing its ability to destroy cancer cells.

Adoptive Cell Therapy:

- In adoptive cell therapy, immune cells (usually T-cells) are extracted from the patient's body, modified or enhanced in the laboratory to be more effective at fighting cancer, and then reintroduced into the body. One such approach is CAR-T (Chimeric Antigen Receptor T-cell) therapy, which has shown great promise in other cancers but is still being researched for its efficacy in pancreatic cancer.

Despite the advances in immunotherapy, pancreatic cancer remains challenging due to its ability to create an immune-suppressive environment within the tumor. However, ongoing research and clinical trials aim to identify which patients may benefit the most from immunotherapy and whether combining it with other treatments can improve outcomes.

2. Targeted Therapy

Targeted therapy uses drugs or other substances to specifically target cancer cells without harming normal cells. Unlike traditional chemotherapy, which kills both healthy and cancerous cells, targeted therapies are designed to target the genetic mutations, proteins, or other molecular abnormalities that drive the growth of cancer cells. These therapies are often less toxic and may be more effective for certain patients.

Targeting Specific Genetic Mutations:

- One of the key aspects of targeted therapy is the identification of genetic mutations in cancer cells that can be targeted with specific drugs. For example, mutations in the KRAS gene, which is common in pancreatic cancer, are a major focus of research. While KRAS mutations have been notoriously difficult to target, new drugs such as Sotorasib and Adagrasib have shown potential in targeting KRAS G12C mutations, a specific subtype of KRAS mutation that may be present in some pancreatic cancers.

HER2-targeted Therapies:

- The HER2 gene, which is implicated in certain cancers like breast and gastric cancers, is sometimes overexpressed in pancreatic cancer as well. Trastuzumab (Herceptin), an HER2-targeted therapy, is being studied for its potential to treat HER2-positive pancreatic cancer, either alone or in combination with chemotherapy.

Angiogenesis Inhibitors:

- Pancreatic tumors require a blood supply to grow and spread. Angiogenesis inhibitors work by blocking the formation of new blood vessels that supply the tumor with oxygen and nutrients. Drugs like Bevacizumab (Avastin), which target vascular endothelial growth factor (VEGF), are being tested in combination with chemotherapy to inhibit tumor growth by cutting off its blood supply.

PARP Inhibitors:

- Poly (ADP-ribose) polymerase (PARP) inhibitors, such as Olaparib (Lynparza), are a type of targeted therapy that block a protein involved in repairing DNA damage in cancer cells. PARP inhibitors have been shown to be effective in cancers with specific genetic mutations, particularly those involving BRCA1 and BRCA2 genes. In pancreatic cancer, patients with hereditary mutations in these genes may benefit from PARP inhibitors, as these cancers are more vulnerable to DNA damage.

While these therapies are still in the investigational stages for pancreatic cancer, clinical trials have shown promising results, particularly for patients with specific genetic mutations or characteristics.

Clinical Trials: What You Should Know

Clinical trials are research studies designed to evaluate new treatments or strategies for managing diseases. They play a crucial role in advancing medical knowledge and discovering more effective ways to treat pancreatic cancer. For patients with pancreatic cancer, participating in a clinical trial may offer access to cutting-edge therapies that are not yet widely available.

1. The Role of Clinical Trials in Cancer Treatment

Clinical trials offer several potential benefits for patients, including access to the latest treatments, more frequent monitoring and care, and contributing to the development of new therapies that may help future patients. Trials are conducted in phases, each designed to answer different scientific questions about safety, dosage, efficacy, and side effects.

- Phase 1 Trials: Focus on evaluating the safety and dosage of a new treatment.
- Phase 2 Trials: Test the efficacy of the treatment and monitor for side effects.
- Phase 3 Trials: Compare the new treatment with the standard treatment to determine which is more effective.
- Phase 4 Trials: Occur after the treatment is approved and monitor its long-term effects and safety.

2. Types of Clinical Trials for Pancreatic Cancer

Clinical trials for pancreatic cancer focus on a variety of therapeutic approaches, including new chemotherapy drugs, novel immunotherapies, targeted therapies, and combination treatments. Trials also explore new methods of delivering treatments, such as localized therapies (e.g., direct injection of drugs into the tumor site) or therapies that boost the effectiveness of existing treatments.

- **Targeted Therapy Trials:** These trials evaluate the effectiveness of specific drugs aimed at molecular targets or genetic mutations in pancreatic cancer, such as KRAS or BRCA1/2 mutations.
- ***Immunotherapy Trials:*** These studies test new immune checkpoint inhibitors, cancer vaccines, and adoptive cell therapies to assess their potential for improving outcomes in pancreatic cancer patients.

- ***Combination Therapy Trials:*** Trials that combine chemotherapy, radiation, immunotherapy, and/or targeted therapy aim to find more effective combinations to treat pancreatic cancer.
- ***Palliative Care Trials***: Focus on improving quality of life by exploring ways to manage pain, improve nutritional status, and alleviate other symptoms.

3. How to Participate in Clinical Trials

Patients interested in participating in clinical trials should discuss this option with their oncologist. Trials have specific eligibility criteria, such as certain genetic profiles, disease stages, or prior treatments, and it is important to understand both the potential benefits and risks. Clinical trial coordinators provide detailed information about the trial design, the treatment being studied, and any potential side effects.

Advances in Personalized Medicine

Personalized medicine refers to tailoring treatment based on the individual characteristics of each patient's cancer, such as genetic mutations or molecular signatures, to optimize effectiveness and minimize unnecessary side effects. In pancreatic cancer, this approach is becoming increasingly important, as each tumor can have a unique genetic profile that influences its behavior and response to treatment.

Genetic Profiling and Biomarkers

- Advances in genetic sequencing technologies have allowed for more precise identification of mutations and alterations in tumor DNA. Testing for mutations in genes such as KRAS, BRCA1/2, p53, and PALB2 can guide treatment decisions. Personalized medicine aims to identify specific biomarkers that can predict how a cancer will respond to targeted therapies, chemotherapy, and immunotherapies.

Liquid Biopsy

- Liquid biopsy is a non-invasive test that analyzes genetic material from a patient's blood, such as circulating tumor DNA (ctDNA), to detect genetic mutations or alterations in pancreatic cancer. Liquid biopsies can help monitor tumor progression, detect minimal residual disease after treatment, and assess the effectiveness of targeted therapies without the need for repeated tissue biopsies.

Patient Stratification

- Personalized medicine also involves stratifying patients into groups based on genetic markers, which allows for the selection of the most effective treatments for each group. For example, patients with specific mutations may be more likely to respond to certain targeted therapies or immunotherapies, leading to more effective treatment regimens and better outcomes.

By integrating genetic testing, molecular profiling, and emerging therapies, personalized medicine is paving the way for more effective and individualized treatment strategies for pancreatic cancer, offering hope for improved survival and quality of life. As research in this field progresses, it holds the potential to significantly transform the management of pancreatic cancer.

Part 3: Living with Pancreatic Cancer

Chapter 7: Nutrition and Digestive Health

Nutrition and digestive health play crucial roles in managing pancreatic cancer and improving the quality of life for individuals with the disease. Pancreatic cancer often impacts the digestive system due to the pancreas' integral role in producing enzymes that aid in digestion and hormones that regulate blood sugar levels. Effective nutritional management can help mitigate complications, address malnutrition, and maintain strength during treatment.

Nutritional Challenges with Pancreatic Cancer

Pancreatic cancer and its treatments frequently lead to significant nutritional challenges, including:

Malnutrition:
- Malnutrition occurs when the body does not get the nutrients it needs to function optimally. In pancreatic cancer, this may result from poor appetite, treatment side effects, or malabsorption of nutrients due to a lack of pancreatic enzymes. Malnutrition can lead to fatigue, reduced immunity, and impaired healing.

Weight Loss:
- Unintentional weight loss is a common concern in pancreatic cancer, often caused by a combination of decreased food intake, malabsorption, and the body's altered metabolism. Maintaining body weight is essential to support overall health and treatment tolerance.

Loss of Muscle Mass (Cachexia):
- Cachexia is a severe form of muscle and weight loss that often occurs in cancer patients, leading to physical weakness and reduced quality of life. Addressing cachexia requires a focus on both caloric and protein intake.

Treatment Side Effects:
- Treatments like chemotherapy or radiation can cause nausea, vomiting, changes in taste, or diarrhea, further complicating nutritional management.

Managing Malabsorption and Weight Loss

Malabsorption occurs when the pancreas does not produce enough enzymes to break down food properly. This leads to undigested food passing through the gastrointestinal tract, resulting in nutrient deficiencies, weight loss, and diarrhea. Management strategies include:

Pancreatic Enzyme Replacement Therapy (PERT):
- PERT involves taking enzyme supplements to help the body digest and absorb nutrients effectively.

These enzymes should be taken with meals and snacks to optimize their effectiveness.

Frequent, Small Meals:
- Eating smaller meals more frequently can help maximize nutrient absorption and reduce the feeling of fullness, which can occur with larger meals.

Nutrient-Dense Foods:
- Focus on foods high in calories and nutrients, such as avocados, nuts, seeds, olive oil, and full-fat dairy products, to address calorie and nutrient needs.

Hydration:
- Staying hydrated is critical, especially for individuals experiencing diarrhea or vomiting. Electrolyte-rich beverages or oral rehydration solutions may be necessary in cases of significant fluid loss.

Monitoring Symptoms:
- Report symptoms like oily stools, diarrhea, or bloating to healthcare providers, as these may indicate insufficient enzyme replacement or other digestive issues.

Foods That Help: A Practical Guide

Certain foods can support digestion, maintain energy levels, and provide essential nutrients:

Proteins:
- Lean meats, poultry, fish, eggs, and dairy products.
- Plant-based proteins like beans, lentils, tofu, and tempeh.

Carbohydrates:
- Whole grains such as brown rice, quinoa, and oatmeal for sustained energy.
- Avoid refined sugars, as they can cause blood sugar spikes.

Healthy Fats:
- Include sources like avocados, olive oil, nuts, seeds, and fatty fish.
- Limit saturated fats and trans fats to avoid unnecessary strain on digestion.

Fruits and Vegetables:
- Opt for cooked or blended options if raw produce causes discomfort.
- Choose nutrient-dense options like spinach, carrots, berries, and bananas.

Probiotics and Prebiotics:
- Probiotics, found in yogurt or fermented foods, support gut health.
- Prebiotic fibers in foods like garlic, onions, and asparagus promote healthy digestion.

Pancreatic Enzymes: Why They're Important and How to Use Them

Pancreatic enzyme replacement therapy is a cornerstone of nutritional management for pancreatic cancer. These enzymes assist in digesting fats, proteins, and carbohydrates, alleviating symptoms of malabsorption and improving nutrient uptake.

Key points about enzyme use include:

Timing and Dosage:
- Enzymes should be taken with every meal or snack to ensure they mix with food in the stomach.
- The dosage depends on the amount of fat in the meal and should be adjusted as per medical advice.

Choosing the Right Supplement:
- There are various enzyme formulations, and healthcare providers can guide the selection of the most appropriate product.

Monitoring Effectiveness:
- Symptoms such as greasy stools or excessive gas may indicate the need for a dosage adjustment or a different enzyme formulation.

Avoiding Acid Interference:
- Some enzymes are sensitive to stomach acid; taking them with acid-reducing medications (like proton pump inhibitors) may improve their effectiveness.

Sample Meal Plans and Recipes

To address nutritional challenges while ensuring variety and enjoyment in meals, consider incorporating the following meal ideas:

Breakfast Options:
- Smoothie with yogurt, almond butter, banana, and a scoop of protein powder.
- Scrambled eggs with sautéed spinach and whole-grain toast.

Lunch Ideas:
- Grilled chicken salad with olive oil dressing and avocado slices.
- Lentil soup with a side of whole-grain bread.

Snacks:
- Greek yogurt with berries and a drizzle of honey.
- A handful of nuts and dried fruit.

Dinner Suggestions:
- Baked salmon with quinoa and roasted vegetables.
- Stir-fried tofu with brown rice and steamed broccoli.

Desserts:
- Mashed sweet potatoes with a sprinkle of cinnamon and a dollop of Greek yogurt.
- Chia seed pudding made with almond milk and fresh fruit toppings.

By addressing nutritional challenges, managing malabsorption, and incorporating practical dietary strategies, individuals with pancreatic cancer can maintain strength, improve digestive health, and enhance their overall well-being. Careful attention to diet, guided by healthcare professionals, plays a vital role in comprehensive cancer care.

Sample 7-Day Meal Plan for Pancreatic Cancer Management

This 7-day meal plan focuses on nutrient-dense foods, small frequent meals, and easily digestible ingredients to address the challenges associated with pancreatic cancer, such as malabsorption, weight loss, and fatigue. It incorporates pancreatic enzyme replacement therapy (PERT) guidance when appropriate.

Day 1
- Breakfast: Scrambled eggs with sautéed spinach, whole-grain toast, and a small glass of fortified almond milk.
- Mid-Morning Snack: Greek yogurt with a tablespoon of chia seeds and a drizzle of honey.
- Lunch: Grilled chicken breast with quinoa and steamed green beans.
- Afternoon Snack: A handful of mixed nuts and dried apricots.
- Dinner: Baked salmon with mashed sweet potatoes and roasted zucchini.
- Evening Snack: Sliced apple with almond butter.

Day 2

- Breakfast: Oatmeal made with almond milk, topped with blueberries, walnuts, and a sprinkle of cinnamon.
- Mid-Morning Snack: A banana and a small handful of sunflower seeds.
- Lunch: Turkey and avocado sandwich on whole-grain bread with a side of carrot sticks.
- Afternoon Snack: Cottage cheese with pineapple chunks.
- Dinner: Stir-fried tofu with brown rice and steamed broccoli.
- Evening Snack: Herbal tea with a slice of whole-grain banana bread.

Day 3

- Breakfast: Smoothie with Greek yogurt, spinach, frozen berries, and a tablespoon of almond butter.
- Mid-Morning Snack: Whole-grain crackers with hummus.
- Lunch: Grilled fish (e.g., cod or haddock) with couscous and roasted asparagus.
- Afternoon Snack: A boiled egg and a slice of whole-grain toast.
- Dinner: Lentil soup with a side of sautéed kale and a slice of whole-grain bread.
- Evening Snack: A small handful of trail mix (nuts and dried fruit).

Day 4

- Breakfast: Omelet with diced tomatoes, mushrooms,

and a sprinkle of low-fat cheese; a slice of whole-grain toast.
- Mid-Morning Snack: A pear and a handful of almonds.
- Lunch: Quinoa salad with grilled chicken, avocado, and mixed greens, dressed with olive oil and lemon juice.
- Afternoon Snack: Yogurt with a teaspoon of ground flaxseeds.
- Dinner: Baked chicken thighs with roasted sweet potatoes and steamed peas.
- Evening Snack: A cup of warm almond milk with a dash of cinnamon.

Day 5
- Breakfast: Whole-grain pancakes topped with almond butter and sliced bananas.
- Mid-Morning Snack: A hard-boiled egg and a handful of cashews.
- Lunch: Grilled shrimp with wild rice and a side of sautéed spinach.
- Afternoon Snack: A smoothie made with almond milk, mango, and chia seeds.
- Dinner: Baked turkey meatballs with whole-grain spaghetti and a light tomato sauce.
- Evening Snack: Fresh strawberries with a dollop of Greek yogurt.

Day 6
- Breakfast: Poached eggs on avocado toast (whole-grain bread).

- Mid-Morning Snack: A small handful of walnuts and dried cranberries.
- Lunch: Baked salmon salad with mixed greens, cherry tomatoes, and olive oil dressing.
- Afternoon Snack: A slice of low-fat cheese with whole-grain crackers.
- Dinner: Grilled chicken with barley and roasted Brussels sprouts.
- Evening Snack: Herbal tea with a slice of oatmeal bar (homemade or low-sugar).

Day 7

- Breakfast: Smoothie bowl with blended frozen bananas, spinach, and almond milk, topped with granola and fresh berries.
- Mid-Morning Snack: A boiled egg and a piece of whole-grain toast.
- Lunch: Tuna salad with olive oil dressing, served with whole-grain crackers.
- Afternoon Snack: A handful of pumpkin seeds and a small apple.
- Dinner: Roasted chicken with quinoa pilaf and a side of sautéed green beans.
- Evening Snack: Warm unsweetened applesauce sprinkled with cinnamon.

Additional Notes

- Portion Sizes: Adjust portion sizes based on individual caloric and nutritional needs.

- Pancreatic Enzymes: Take pancreatic enzyme supplements (if prescribed) with meals and snacks to ensure proper nutrient absorption.
- Hydration: Include plenty of fluids throughout the day, such as water, herbal teas, or clear broths.
- Customizations: Substitute ingredients as needed to accommodate preferences, dietary restrictions, or availability.

Chapter 8: Exercise and Physical Activity

The Role of Exercise in Pancreatic Cancer Care

Exercise plays a critical role in maintaining physical and mental well-being for individuals diagnosed with pancreatic cancer. While the intensity and type of exercise may vary depending on the stage of cancer, treatment status, and overall health, incorporating physical activity can offer multiple benefits.

Benefits of Physical Activity

1. Improved Energy Levels: Regular movement helps combat fatigue, a common side effect of cancer treatments like chemotherapy and radiation therapy.
2. Enhanced Muscle Strength: Exercise can counteract muscle loss (cachexia) and improve functional strength.
3. Mood and Mental Health Support: Physical activity releases endorphins, reducing symptoms of anxiety and depression.
4. Better Digestion: Light exercises, like walking, can promote gastrointestinal motility and reduce bloating or discomfort.

5. Immune Function Support: Moderate exercise may enhance immune system efficiency.
6. Bone Health: Weight-bearing exercises help combat bone density loss caused by treatment or malnutrition.
7. Improved Circulation: Regular activity prevents blood clots, a risk associated with pancreatic cancer.

Types of Physical Activity

1. Aerobic Exercise: Activities like walking, swimming, or cycling improve cardiovascular health and stamina.

- Recommended: 20–30 minutes, 3–5 times per week.
- Adjust intensity to tolerance; even slow walking is beneficial.

2. *Strength Training:* Light resistance training can maintain or rebuild muscle mass.

- Examples: Bodyweight exercises, resistance bands, or light weights.
- Frequency: 2–3 times per week with a day of rest in between.

3. Flexibility and Balance: Stretching exercises improve mobility and reduce the risk of falls.

- Yoga or Pilates can combine flexibility with mindfulness.
- Stretch major muscle groups daily for 10–15 minutes.

4. *Breathing Exercises:* Controlled breathing techniques, often part of yoga or tai chi, improve lung function and reduce stress.

Designing a Personalized Exercise Plan

1. Consult a Healthcare Provider: Before starting, discuss with an oncologist or physical therapist to ensure safety and appropriateness.
2. Consider Treatment Effects: Modify activities to accommodate fatigue, nausea, or neuropathy caused by treatments.
3. Start Slowly: Gradually increase the intensity and duration of exercises.
4. Listen to the Body: Rest when needed and avoid pushing through extreme fatigue or pain.
5. Hydration and Nutrition: Ensure adequate fluid intake and balanced meals to support physical activity.

Sample Weekly Exercise Plan for Individuals with Pancreatic Cancer

Day 1: 20-minute light walk + 10 minutes of gentle stretching.

Day 2: 15 minutes of yoga or tai chi + resistance band exercises (arms and shoulders).

Day 3: Rest or light breathing exercises.

Day 4: 25-minute swim or cycling at a moderate pace.

Day 5: 20-minute walk + core-strength exercises (e.g., seated leg lifts).

Day 6: Stretching routine + 10 minutes of balance exercises.
Day 7: Rest or light physical activity, like gardening or slow walking.

Safety Tips for Exercising During Treatment

1. Monitor Symptoms: Stop exercising if you experience dizziness, shortness of breath, or pain.
2. Avoid Heavy Lifting: Especially if surgery or advanced disease has impacted abdominal strength.
3. Be Mindful of Neuropathy: Use supportive footwear to prevent falls if experiencing tingling or numbness.
4. Protect Surgical Sites: Avoid movements that strain areas affected by surgery.

By integrating tailored physical activity into daily routines, patients can enhance their overall quality of life and improve their ability to manage the physical and emotional challenges of pancreatic cancer. Regular check-ins with healthcare professionals ensure these exercises remain safe and effective throughout treatment and recovery.

Chapter 9: Coping with Emotional and Psychological Impact

The diagnosis and management of pancreatic cancer extend beyond physical health; the emotional and psychological challenges can be profound. Understanding and addressing these aspects are essential for holistic care and overall well-being. The following sections explore the emotional toll, common psychological responses, and effective strategies to build resilience and find support.

Understanding the Emotional Toll

Pancreatic cancer is a life-altering condition that often evokes a range of intense emotions. The emotional impact may stem from various factors, including:

Uncertainty:
- The complexity of treatment options and potential outcomes can create a sense of unpredictability.

Loss of Control:
- Physical changes, medical procedures, and disruptions to daily life can lead to feelings of helplessness.

Changes in Roles and Relationships:

- Shifts in responsibilities and dynamics within personal and professional relationships can be challenging to navigate.

Financial and Logistical Strains:

- Costs associated with treatment and adjustments to work or living arrangements can exacerbate emotional stress.

Anxiety, Depression, and Fear

Emotional distress often manifests as anxiety, depression, and fear. Understanding these responses is vital to implementing effective coping mechanisms.

Anxiety:

- Anxiety may arise from concerns about disease progression, treatment side effects, or future uncertainties. Symptoms can include restlessness, difficulty concentrating, and physical manifestations such as rapid heartbeat or shallow breathing.

Depression:

- Feelings of sadness, hopelessness, or a lack of motivation may signal depression. It can interfere with daily functioning and reduce the effectiveness of coping strategies.

Fear:

- Fear of the unknown, potential pain, or changes

in quality of life is a natural response. It may also lead to avoidance behaviors, such as hesitating to seek treatment or support.

Cumulative Stress:
- The combination of physical symptoms, treatment demands, and emotional challenges can lead to burnout or overwhelming stress if not addressed.

Building Resilience and Positivity

Resilience refers to the ability to adapt to adversity and maintain mental well-being. While emotional responses to pancreatic cancer are natural, resilience-building strategies can help manage these challenges effectively.

Acceptance:
- Acknowledging emotions and the reality of the situation is the first step toward proactive coping. Denial or suppression of emotions may delay necessary actions.

Mindfulness and Relaxation Techniques:
- Practices such as meditation, deep breathing, and progressive muscle relaxation can reduce anxiety and promote a sense of calm.

Focus on Small Achievements:
- Setting manageable goals, such as completing a light exercise routine or engaging in a hobby, can boost self-esteem and positivity.

Maintaining Routine:
- Structure and predictability in daily activities provide a sense of normalcy and control.

Professional Support:
- Psychologists, counselors, or social workers specializing in oncology can offer tools to manage emotions effectively. Cognitive-behavioral therapy (CBT) and other evidence-based approaches may be particularly helpful.

Finding Support: Family, Friends, and Support Groups

A robust support system is a key component of emotional well-being. Building and maintaining connections with others can provide comfort, encouragement, and practical assistance.

Family and Friends:
- Communication: Openly discussing emotions, needs, and expectations fosters understanding and strengthens relationships.
- Involvement: Involving loved ones in appointments, treatment planning, or daily routines can reduce feelings of isolation.

Support Groups:
- Shared Experiences: Connecting with others facing similar challenges can provide a sense of community and validation.

- Educational Value: Many groups offer insights into coping strategies, treatment advancements, and resources.
- Accessibility: Support groups are available in person and online, making them a flexible option.

Community Resources:
- Organizations dedicated to cancer care often provide emotional support services, including helplines, workshops, and peer counseling.
- Faith-based or cultural groups may also offer comfort aligned with personal values.

Healthcare Team:
- Oncologists, nurses, and palliative care specialists can address concerns and recommend resources tailored to individual needs.

Coping with the emotional and psychological impact of pancreatic cancer requires a multifaceted approach. Acknowledging and addressing the emotional toll, building resilience, and utilizing support systems can significantly improve quality of life. Emotional well-being is an integral part of comprehensive cancer care, and prioritizing it is essential for managing the journey effectively.

Chapter 10: Palliative Care and Symptom Management

Palliative care plays an essential role in the management of pancreatic cancer, focusing on relieving symptoms and improving the quality of life for individuals at any stage of the disease. This chapter explores the scope of palliative care, techniques for managing common symptoms, and strategies to enhance overall well-being.

The Role of Palliative Care at Any Stage

Palliative care is a specialized medical approach aimed at improving comfort and addressing the physical, emotional, and psychological burdens associated with serious illnesses. It is not limited to end-of-life care and can be integrated alongside curative or life-prolonging treatments.

Goals of Palliative Care:
- Alleviation of symptoms such as pain, nausea, and fatigue.
- Support for emotional and psychological health.
- Assistance with decision-making regarding treatment options.

- Enhancement of quality of life regardless of disease stage.

Palliative Care Team:
- The care team often includes physicians, nurses, social workers, dietitians, and spiritual counselors who work collaboratively to address diverse needs.

Early Integration:
- Studies show that incorporating palliative care early in the treatment process can lead to better symptom control, reduced stress, and improved outcomes.

Pain Management Techniques

Pain is a common symptom in pancreatic cancer due to tumor pressure on surrounding organs or nerve involvement. Effective pain management requires a tailored approach.

Medications:
- Non-Opioids: Nonsteroidal anti inflammatory drugs (NSAIDs) and acetaminophen are used for mild to moderate pain.
- Opioids: Medications such as morphine or oxycodone are prescribed for moderate to severe pain. Dosages are carefully adjusted to minimize side effects.
- Adjuvant Medications: Antidepressants or anticonvulsants may be used to address nerve pain (neuropathy).

Nerve Blocks:

- Celiac plexus blocks involve injecting an anesthetic or alcohol-based solution near the nerves transmitting pain from the pancreas, providing significant relief in some cases.

Radiation Therapy:

- Targeted radiation can shrink tumors causing pain, alleviating pressure on nearby tissues.

Non-Pharmacological Techniques:

- Physical Therapy: Gentle exercises and stretching can reduce muscle tension contributing to pain.
- Complementary Therapies: Acupuncture, massage, and relaxation techniques such as yoga or mindfulness meditation may provide additional relief.

Dealing with Fatigue, Nausea, and Digestive Issues

Managing common symptoms effectively is a key component of palliative care.

Fatigue:

- Energy Conservation: Prioritize activities, rest between tasks, and delegate responsibilities when possible.
- Address Underlying Causes: Fatigue may stem from anemia, poor nutrition, or treatment side effects.

Treating these underlying issues can help mitigate exhaustion.

- Exercise: Light physical activity, such as walking, can boost energy levels and reduce fatigue.

Nausea and Vomiting:

- Medications: Anti-nausea drugs (antiemetics) such as ondansetron or metoclopramide are commonly used to control symptoms.
- Dietary Adjustments: Small, frequent meals and avoiding strong smells or greasy foods can reduce nausea triggers.
- Hydration: Maintaining fluid intake helps prevent dehydration caused by vomiting.

Digestive Issues:

- Malabsorption: Pancreatic enzyme replacement therapy (PERT) can improve digestion and nutrient absorption.
- Diarrhea: Anti-diarrheal medications, such as loperamide, and dietary adjustments can manage symptoms.
- Constipation: Adequate hydration, dietary fiber, and stool softeners can help alleviate constipation, which may be exacerbated by opioid use.

Enhancing Quality of Life

Palliative care goes beyond symptom control, addressing the broader aspects of well-being to enhance overall quality of life.

Emotional and Psychological Support:
- Access to counseling or therapy can help individuals cope with the emotional challenges of living with pancreatic cancer.
- Stress-reduction techniques, such as mindfulness or art therapy, can provide emotional relief.

Nutritional Support:
- Tailored meal plans focusing on nutrient-dense, easy-to-digest foods can improve strength and overall health.
- A registered dietitian can provide guidance on managing appetite changes and meeting caloric needs.

Social Support:
- Maintaining connections with family and friends provides emotional strength and reduces feelings of isolation.
- Support groups or community resources can create a sense of shared understanding and camaraderie.

Spiritual and Existential Care:
- Addressing spiritual needs, whether through religious practices or personal reflection, can bring comfort and meaning.

- Palliative care teams often include chaplains or spiritual counselors to provide guidance.

Care Coordination:
- Palliative care specialists work with oncologists and other medical professionals to ensure seamless integration of symptom management with ongoing treatments.

Palliative care and symptom management are integral components of comprehensive care for pancreatic cancer. By addressing physical symptoms, emotional challenges, and quality-of-life concerns, palliative care ensures a holistic approach to treatment that prioritizes comfort and dignity at every stage of the disease. Early integration and effective communication with the care team can significantly enhance well-being and overall outcomes.

Part 4: Navigating the Journey After Diagnosis

Chapter 11: Building Your Healthcare Team

A multidisciplinary healthcare team is essential in managing pancreatic cancer, as it ensures that all aspects of care—medical, physical, emotional, and logistical—are addressed. Understanding the roles of key professionals, knowing what questions to ask, and advocating for one's needs are critical for optimizing care and outcomes.

Roles of Oncologists, Surgeons, and Specialists

Effective care for pancreatic cancer often involves collaboration among several medical professionals, each contributing specialized expertise.

Oncologists:

- Medical Oncologists: Focus on systemic treatments like chemotherapy, targeted therapy, or immunotherapy. They coordinate treatment plans and monitor treatment effectiveness.
- Radiation Oncologists: Specialize in using radiation therapy to shrink tumors or manage symptoms, such as pain.

- Role in Follow-Up: Oncologists play a central role in long-term management, including monitoring for recurrence or side effects.

Surgeons:
- Surgical Oncologists: Specialize in operations like the Whipple procedure, distal pancreatectomy, or total pancreatectomy when surgery is an option.
- Role in Diagnosis: Surgeons may also perform biopsies or exploratory surgeries to aid in diagnosis or staging.

Gastroenterologists:
- Experts in digestive health who address complications such as malabsorption, jaundice, or bile duct obstruction. They may place stents or perform procedures like endoscopic retrograde cholangiopancreatography (ERCP).

Palliative Care Specialists:
- Focus on symptom management, including pain relief, fatigue, and psychological support, at any stage of the disease.

Dietitians:
- Provide guidance on nutrition tailored to pancreatic cancer, addressing weight loss, malabsorption, and energy needs.

Nurses and Nurse Navigators:
- Coordinate care, provide education about treatments,

and offer practical support during medical appointments and procedures.

Psychologists and Social Workers:
- Address emotional, psychological, and social challenges, helping to navigate logistical and financial aspects of care.

Genetic Counselors:
- Evaluate genetic predispositions that may influence treatment options or the need for family screening.

Pharmacists:
- Help manage medications, including chemotherapy drugs, pain relievers, and supplements, while monitoring for potential interactions.

Questions to Ask Your Doctor

Open and clear communication with the healthcare team is essential for informed decision-making. The following are key questions to consider during consultations:

About the Diagnosis:
- What type of pancreatic cancer do I have, and what is its stage?
- Are there biomarkers or genetic tests that could guide treatment?

About Treatment Options:
- What are the recommended treatments, and what are

their goals (curative, palliative, or symptom management)?
- What are the potential benefits and risks of each treatment option?
- Are there clinical trials available?

About Side Effects and Management:
- What side effects should I expect, and how can they be managed?
- How will treatments affect my daily life, including work, exercise, and social activities?

About the Care Team:
- Who will coordinate my care, and how can I reach them in case of emergencies?
- Will I need referrals to additional specialists or services?

About Support Services:
- Are there resources available for emotional or psychological support?
- What nutritional guidance is recommended?

About Long-Term Outlook:
- What follow-up care will be required after treatment?
- How will recurrence or progression be monitored?

Advocating for Your Needs

Advocacy is an essential skill in ensuring that medical care aligns with personal preferences, values, and goals. Here are strategies to effectively advocate for needs:

Educating Yourself:
- Stay informed about pancreatic cancer, its treatments, and emerging advances. Reliable resources include peer-reviewed journals, cancer organizations, and patient advocacy groups.

Preparing for Appointments:
- Create a list of questions or concerns before appointments. Bringing a notebook or using a smartphone to record discussions can help with retention of complex information.

Involving Others:
- Enlist a trusted friend or family member to attend appointments as an advocate. They can take notes, ask additional questions, and provide support.

Communicating Clearly:
- Express preferences and concerns openly, whether about treatment options, side effects, or logistical challenges. Healthcare providers rely on clear communication to tailor care effectively.

Seeking Second Opinions:
- It is acceptable and often encouraged to seek a

second opinion, especially when considering major decisions like surgery or enrollment in clinical trials.

Utilizing Resources:
- Many hospitals and cancer centers have patient advocates, nurse navigators, or social workers who can assist in resolving issues, accessing resources, or navigating insurance.

Maintaining Records:
- Keep an organized record of medical history, test results, treatment plans, and medication lists. This facilitates smooth communication across multiple providers.

Building a comprehensive healthcare team and actively participating in care are fundamental components of effective pancreatic cancer management. Each member of the team brings specialized expertise, contributing to a well-rounded approach to treatment. By asking the right questions, advocating for needs, and fostering collaborative relationships, individuals can ensure they receive personalized, high-quality care that aligns with their goals and circumstances.

Chapter 12: Practical Considerations

Effective management of pancreatic cancer extends beyond medical treatment, encompassing financial, legal, and lifestyle adjustments. Addressing these practical aspects proactively can help alleviate stress and ensure a more seamless care experience. This chapter explores insurance and financial considerations, adapting to changes in daily life, and planning for future care and legal matters.

Understanding Insurance and Financial Assistance

Cancer care can be financially burdensome, involving costs related to diagnostics, treatments, medications, and supportive care. Understanding insurance options and seeking financial assistance can mitigate these challenges.

Health Insurance Coverage:
- Review policy details to understand what is covered, including diagnostic tests, treatments (chemotherapy, radiation, surgery), medications, and follow-up care.
- Determine out-of-pocket costs, such as co-pays, deductibles, and maximum out-of-pocket limits.

Pre-authorization and Referrals:

- Some insurance plans require prior authorization for treatments or referrals to specialists. It is essential to ensure these steps are completed to avoid delays or denied claims.

Financial Assistance Programs:

- Many hospitals and cancer centers have financial counselors who can assist in navigating payment plans, discounts, or charity care programs.
- Organizations like the Pancreatic Cancer Action Network, American Cancer Society, and CancerCare offer resources and grants to assist with treatment-related expenses.

Government Assistance:

- Programs such as Medicaid, Medicare, or Social Security Disability Insurance (SSDI) may provide support for eligible individuals.
- Supplemental Security Income (SSI) may be available for those with limited income and resources.

Managing Unexpected Costs:

- Include transportation, lodging (for treatment at distant centers), and caregiver expenses in budgeting plans.
- Nonprofit organizations often provide travel and lodging assistance for cancer patients.

Work, Family, and Lifestyle Adjustments

Managing pancreatic cancer often necessitates changes in work and family life, as well as adjustments to daily routines.

Workplace Considerations:

- Medical Leave: Understand rights under laws such as the Family and Medical Leave Act (FMLA), which provides eligible employees with unpaid, job-protected leave.
- Workplace Accommodations: Flexible schedules, reduced hours, or remote work options can help balance treatment and employment.
- Disability Benefits: Short-term or long-term disability insurance may provide income replacement if work is temporarily or permanently affected.

Family Roles and Responsibilities:

- Adjustments in household roles may be necessary to accommodate physical limitations or treatment schedules.
- Clear communication among family members about needs and expectations can minimize stress and foster teamwork.

Lifestyle Modifications:

- Energy Management: Incorporate rest periods into daily routines to manage fatigue effectively.
- Dietary Adjustments: Follow a nutrition plan tailored to pancreatic cancer management, as discussed in Chapter 7.

- Physical Activity: Engage in light exercises, such as walking or yoga, to maintain physical strength and reduce stress.

Childcare and Dependent Care:
- For those with children or dependents, planning for caregiving support can reduce the emotional and logistical strain.
- Explore resources for temporary or long-term care assistance through community organizations or social services.

Advance Care Planning and Legal Considerations

Advance care planning ensures that medical and personal preferences are honored, while legal preparedness provides peace of mind and clarity for families and caregivers.

Advance Directives:
- Living Will: Documents preferences for medical care, including resuscitation, life support, and other interventions.
- Durable Power of Attorney for Healthcare: Appoints a trusted individual to make medical decisions if one is unable to do so.

Financial and Legal Documents:
- Durable Power of Attorney for Finances: Authorizes someone to manage financial matters, including paying bills and handling insurance claims.
- Will and Estate Planning: Ensures that personal assets are distributed according to one's wishes and minimizes disputes.

Palliative and Hospice Care Preferences:
- Clearly outline preferences for palliative care or hospice care if needed, including locations (home, hospice facility, hospital).

Organizing Important Documents:
- Compile and store medical records, insurance policies, advance directives, and legal documents in a secure and accessible location.
- Share the location and details with trusted family members or legal representatives.

Accessing Legal Resources:
- Seek guidance from attorneys or nonprofit organizations specializing in healthcare law and cancer-related legal issues.
- Many hospitals provide access to legal aid services for patients and their families.

Practical considerations, such as navigating financial challenges, adjusting to lifestyle changes, and preparing for future care, are integral to comprehensive cancer management. Addressing these aspects systematically and proactively can reduce stress, foster stability, and ensure that medical and personal priorities are respected throughout the journey. These steps provide a foundation for focusing on treatment and well-being with greater confidence and peace of mind.

Chapter 13: Staying Informed and Proactive

Effective post-treatment management of pancreatic cancer requires ongoing vigilance, clear communication with healthcare providers, and staying informed about emerging research and treatment options. This chapter outlines essential practices for health monitoring, symptom tracking, and keeping up-to-date with scientific advancements to ensure proactive and informed care.

Monitoring Your Health Post-Treatment

After treatment, regular monitoring is critical to detect potential recurrence, manage late effects of therapy, and maintain overall health.

Scheduled Follow-Ups:

- Frequency: Follow-up schedules are typically determined by the healthcare team based on the type of treatment received and the individual's health status. Appointments may range from every 3–6 months initially to annual visits over time.
- Assessments: Follow-up visits may include physical examinations, imaging studies (CT, MRI, or PET scans), and laboratory tests (e.g., tumor markers like CA 19-9) to monitor for recurrence.

- Coordination: Ensure that all relevant specialists—oncologists, gastroenterologists, and primary care physicians—are involved in follow-up care.

Managing Long-Term Side Effects:
- Address lingering or late-onset side effects of treatment, such as fatigue, neuropathy, digestive issues, or hormonal imbalances.
- Pancreatic enzyme replacement therapy (PERT) or insulin therapy may be required for those who have undergone surgical procedures affecting pancreatic function.

Preventive Health:
- Focus on overall health maintenance, including managing comorbid conditions like diabetes or cardiovascular disease.
- Regular screening for other cancers or illnesses based on individual risk factors is essential.

Tracking Symptoms and Reporting Changes

Proactive symptom tracking and timely reporting of concerns can facilitate early detection of complications or recurrence, enabling prompt intervention.

Common Symptoms to Monitor:
- Digestive Issues: New or worsening nausea,

vomiting, diarrhea, or jaundice may indicate complications or disease progression.
- Unexplained Pain: Abdominal or back pain can be a sign of recurrence or other conditions requiring medical attention.
- Weight Changes: Sudden, unintentional weight loss may suggest malabsorption, metabolic changes, or disease recurrence.

Keeping Records:
- Maintain a detailed symptom journal noting the nature, frequency, and severity of symptoms. Include any potential triggers or patterns.
- Document dietary intake, medication use, and energy levels to identify trends that may warrant medical attention.

Communication with Healthcare Providers:
- Report new or concerning symptoms promptly, even between scheduled visits. Early intervention can prevent complications and improve outcomes.
- Use patient portals or direct contact with care teams to streamline communication.

Staying Updated on New Research

Ongoing advancements in pancreatic cancer research may offer access to improved treatments, emerging therapies, and innovative approaches to care.

Sources of Reliable Information:

- Scientific Journals: Peer-reviewed publications provide the most credible and detailed information about new findings in cancer care.
- Medical Institutions and Cancer Centers: Leading institutions such as the National Cancer Institute (NCI), American Society of Clinical Oncology (ASCO), and Pancreatic Cancer Action Network regularly publish updates on research and clinical trials.
- Conferences and Webinars: Events organized by professional societies are excellent platforms for learning about cutting-edge developments.

Participating in Clinical Trials:

- Explore eligibility for clinical trials investigating novel treatments, such as targeted therapy, immunotherapy, or combination regimens.
- Trials offer access to experimental therapies while contributing to the advancement of science.

Emerging Areas of Research:

- Genomic and Biomarker Studies: Advances in genetic profiling are paving the way for personalized medicine, enabling treatments tailored to specific tumor characteristics.
- Immunotherapy: Continued research into immune checkpoint inhibitors and other immunotherapies holds promise for expanding treatment options.

- Early Detection Techniques: Development of biomarkers and imaging tools aims to improve early diagnosis and intervention.

Engaging with Advocacy and Support Organizations:
- Organizations focused on pancreatic cancer research often provide newsletters, webinars, and updates to keep patients and families informed.
- Advocacy groups also facilitate connections to experts and resources for navigating treatment and survivorship.

Staying informed and proactive post-treatment is a cornerstone of long-term management for pancreatic cancer. Regular monitoring, diligent symptom tracking, and awareness of new research ensure that individuals remain empowered to address changes in health and take advantage of advances in care. Collaboration with healthcare providers and access to reliable information are key to navigating this evolving landscape and optimizing health outcomes.

Part 5: Resources and Inspiration

Chapter 14: Real Stories, Real Strength

While pancreatic cancer presents significant challenges, the experiences of those who have navigated this journey offer valuable lessons in resilience and adaptation. Survivors and caregivers alike provide insights into overcoming difficulties and finding strength in the face of adversity. This chapter highlights illustrative accounts to shed light on these experiences, serving as an inspiration and guide for others.

Accounts from Pancreatic Cancer Survivors

1. Navigating Complex Treatments

One survivor, a retired teacher, shared how early detection during a routine medical examination led to a successful Whipple procedure. The recovery was arduous, involving dietary changes and managing fatigue, but with the support of her care team and adherence to post-surgical recommendations, she resumed an active lifestyle. Her experience underscores the importance of timely medical attention and a proactive approach to health.

2. Managing Long-Term Effects

A young professional diagnosed at an advanced stage underwent chemotherapy and participated in a clinical trial for targeted therapy. Though side effects like neuropathy and weight loss posed challenges, regular consultations with dietitians and physical therapists helped him regain strength. His story highlights the role of supportive care in improving quality of life during and after treatment.

3. Finding New Purpose

A retired engineer who achieved remission through surgery and chemotherapy turned his focus to raising awareness about pancreatic cancer. His advocacy efforts involved speaking at community events and supporting others through patient networks. He emphasized the therapeutic value of channeling energy into meaningful causes.

Survivors of pancreatic cancer exemplify determination and adaptability. Their experiences often highlight the importance of comprehensive care, early intervention, and a proactive mindset.

Navigating the Diagnosis and Treatment:

- Many survivors emphasize the value of early and accurate diagnosis in shaping treatment outcomes.
- The role of multidisciplinary care teams, including surgeons, oncologists, dietitians, and mental health professionals, is consistently recognized as pivotal.
- Survivors often credit tailored treatment plans, including combinations of surgery, chemotherapy, and lifestyle modifications, for their successful management of the disease.

Adjusting to Lifestyle Changes:

- Post-treatment, survivors frequently highlight the

importance of ongoing dietary adjustments, use of pancreatic enzyme replacement therapy (PERT), and managing long-term side effects like fatigue or neuropathy.
* Maintaining physical activity, even at a reduced intensity, is commonly mentioned as a way to improve energy levels and emotional well-being.

Finding Resilience in Challenges:
* Survivors often report that building a strong support system of family, friends, and healthcare providers played a crucial role in their journey.
* Many discuss how engaging with support groups, advocacy organizations, or counseling helped them cope with the psychological challenges of a cancer diagnosis.

Lessons Learned from Caregivers

1. Balancing Care and Support

A caregiver who supported her spouse through late-stage pancreatic cancer shared how she juggled appointments, symptom management, and household responsibilities. She emphasized the importance of creating a structured schedule and seeking help from extended family and friends when needed. Her story illustrates the significance of shared responsibilities in caregiving.

2. Advocating for Better Care

The son of a pancreatic cancer patient played a key role in exploring treatment options, seeking second opinions, and coordinating with specialists. His persistence ensured access to a clinical trial that improved his parent's quality of life. This case highlights the critical role of informed advocacy in cancer care.

3. Coping with Emotional Strain

A caregiver who supported her sibling during treatment recounted the emotional toll of the experience. Regular counseling sessions and participation in a caregiver support group helped her manage stress and grief. Her journey underscores the importance of self-care and emotional support for caregivers.

Caregivers provide invaluable support throughout the cancer journey, often managing logistical, emotional, and physical demands. Their insights shed light on how to provide effective and compassionate care.

Adapting to the Caregiving Role:

- Caregivers often describe the initial adjustment period as challenging, requiring a quick understanding of the disease, treatment protocols, and the needs of the individual with cancer.
- Many recommend establishing a clear routine that accommodates medical appointments, symptom management, and personal caregiving responsibilities.

Emphasizing Communication:

- Open, honest communication with healthcare providers is frequently mentioned as critical for ensuring the patient receives optimal care.

- Caregivers also stress the importance of discussing preferences and concerns with the individual they are supporting to align on care goals.

Self-Care for Caregivers:
- A recurring theme is the need for caregivers to prioritize their own well-being, balancing caregiving duties with self-care to prevent burnout.
- Engaging with peer support groups or seeking professional counseling is often cited as beneficial for maintaining emotional health.

Practical Strategies for Management:
- Caregivers highlight the importance of staying organized, using tools such as calendars, medication trackers, and symptom logs to streamline care.
- Many emphasize the value of learning about palliative care options early to address symptoms like pain and fatigue effectively.

Advocacy and Empowerment:
- Advocating for the best possible care, whether by asking detailed questions during appointments or seeking second opinions, is often described as a crucial caregiver responsibility.
- Several caregivers mention becoming active in cancer advocacy groups to contribute to broader awareness and support initiatives.

The experiences of pancreatic cancer survivors and caregivers provide a deeper understanding of the realities of managing this challenging disease. Their stories underscore the importance of resilience, adaptability, and proactive care, offering valuable lessons for individuals navigating similar circumstances. By learning from these accounts, others can find inspiration and practical guidance for their own journeys, reaffirming that strength and support are central to overcoming the challenges of pancreatic cancer.

Chapter 15: Advocacy and Raising Awareness

Advocacy plays a vital role in improving outcomes for individuals affected by pancreatic cancer. It not only helps raise awareness of the disease but also fosters advancements in research, treatment, and support systems. Advocacy efforts are often driven by patients, families, healthcare professionals, and organizations dedicated to making a difference. This chapter discusses how to engage in advocacy and support the global fight against pancreatic cancer.

Joining the Fight Against Pancreatic Cancer

Advocacy starts with a commitment to raising awareness about the disease, reducing stigma, and encouraging timely detection and treatment. These efforts can take various forms and have significant impacts at local, national, and global levels.

Raising Awareness:
- Public Education Campaigns: Efforts to educate communities about the symptoms, risk factors, and importance of early detection help combat low awareness associated with pancreatic cancer.
- World Pancreatic Cancer Day: Observed annually, this day unites people worldwide in spreading

awareness and emphasizing the need for research and support. Participating in events or campaigns is an effective way to contribute.

- Leveraging Media Platforms: Social media, blogs, and local news outlets can be powerful tools to share verified information and personal or general advocacy messages.

Engaging with Local and National Advocacy Groups:
- Organizations like the Pancreatic Cancer Action Network (PanCAN) and similar groups worldwide offer structured programs for advocacy, including petitioning for healthcare reforms and research funding.
- Joining these groups provides access to resources, training, and opportunities to amplify the impact of one's efforts.

Advocacy in Healthcare Policy:
- Advocacy initiatives often focus on improving healthcare policies, such as increasing funding for cancer research, ensuring equitable access to treatments, and expanding coverage for essential therapies.
- Collaborating with policymakers and healthcare leaders can drive systemic changes that benefit a wider population.

Supporting Research and Fundraising

Supporting research is essential to uncovering new treatments, improving survival rates, and enhancing the quality of life for those affected by pancreatic cancer. Fundraising is a practical and impactful way to fuel this progress.

The Role of Research in Advancing Care:
- Research efforts focus on understanding the biological mechanisms of pancreatic cancer, developing early diagnostic tools, and creating innovative therapies such as immunotherapy and targeted treatments.
- Participation in clinical trials is a form of direct contribution to research and provides valuable data that informs future treatment approaches.

Ways to Support Research:
- Donations: Financial contributions to reputable cancer research institutions or specific studies help fund groundbreaking investigations.
- Volunteering: Assisting with research awareness events or clinical trial recruitment can significantly support ongoing studies.
- Educational Outreach: Promoting the importance of scientific research to communities and decision-makers helps garner broader support and funding.

Effective Fundraising Strategies:
- Community Events: Hosting events such as walks,

marathons, or bake sales raises funds while spreading awareness.

- Corporate Partnerships: Collaborating with businesses to sponsor events or match donations can amplify efforts.
- Online Campaigns: Crowdfunding platforms and social media fundraising drives allow for widespread participation and contributions.

Recognizing Contributions:
- Highlighting successful research outcomes and acknowledging contributors helps sustain enthusiasm and engagement. Transparency about the use of funds builds trust and encourages ongoing support.

The Power of Collective Action

Advocacy and fundraising thrive on collaboration. Partnering with advocacy groups, healthcare institutions, and research organizations strengthens efforts and broadens the reach of initiatives. Additionally, collective action unites diverse voices to create a stronger impact in the fight against pancreatic cancer.

Building Networks:
- Networking with other advocates and organizations fosters a sense of community and shared purpose.
- Partnerships enable access to broader audiences and additional resources.

Celebrating Progress:
- Highlighting milestones in awareness campaigns, fundraising achievements, or research breakthroughs reinforces the importance of advocacy.
- Success stories encourage continued participation and investment in advocacy efforts.

Advocacy and fundraising are powerful tools in the fight against pancreatic cancer. By raising awareness, supporting research, and engaging with communities and policymakers, individuals and organizations can make meaningful contributions to improving outcomes for those affected by this disease. Collective action, driven by informed and passionate advocacy, holds the potential to transform the future of pancreatic cancer care and research.

Conclusion

Pancreatic cancer presents a significant challenge, both medically and emotionally, for patients and their families. However, with the right knowledge, resources, and support, it is possible to navigate the complexities of diagnosis, treatment, and care. The journey requires not only medical intervention but also emotional resilience, lifestyle adjustments, and an understanding of the disease's impact on daily life.

This guide has aimed to provide clear, evidence-based insights into the medical, nutritional, and psychological aspects of pancreatic cancer. From understanding the fundamentals of pancreatic cancer, its types, and risk factors, to exploring treatment options, symptom management, and emotional support strategies, each chapter serves as a building block toward a holistic approach to managing the disease.

The key takeaway is that, while pancreatic cancer is undeniably a serious illness, medical advancements continue to improve survival rates and quality of life. Early detection, personalized treatment plans, and the incorporation of physical and emotional well-being into care are central to achieving the best possible outcomes. Patients and caregivers alike can find empowerment in making informed decisions, advocating for the best care, and utilizing the support networks available to them.

Ultimately, moving forward with confidence and a proactive mindset is essential. Stay informed, engage with healthcare providers, and seek support from family, friends, and professional networks. By combining treatment with a focus on overall well-being, individuals with pancreatic cancer can maintain a quality of life and continue to face the challenges ahead with hope and strength.

Appendices

The appendices provide supplementary resources to enhance understanding, clarify complex topics, and connect readers with support systems. This section aims to serve as a quick reference guide for terms, common concerns, and practical resources related to pancreatic cancer.

Glossary of Terms

To navigate the medical and technical aspects of pancreatic cancer, understanding key terminology is essential. Below is a glossary of frequently encountered terms:

- Adenocarcinoma: The most common type of pancreatic cancer, originating in the exocrine cells of the pancreas.

- Biopsy: A procedure in which a small tissue sample is taken for examination under a microscope to determine the presence of cancer cells.

- Chemotherapy: The use of drugs to destroy or inhibit the growth of cancer cells.

- Exocrine Tumor: A tumor arising from the exocrine cells of the pancreas, which produce digestive enzymes.

- Endocrine Tumor: A tumor originating in the hormone-producing (endocrine) cells of the pancreas, such as insulinomas.

- Palliative Care: A specialized form of medical care focused on relieving symptoms and improving the quality of life for individuals with serious illnesses.

- Whipple Procedure: A surgical operation to remove part of the pancreas, the duodenum, and other nearby tissues, often performed for pancreatic cancer.

Advanced Glossary Terms for Pancreatic Cancer

Adjuvant Therapy
- Treatment given after the primary treatment (e.g., surgery) to reduce the risk of cancer recurrence, including chemotherapy or radiation therapy.

Biliary Obstruction
- A blockage in the bile ducts, often caused by tumors, which can lead to jaundice.

Biomarkers
- Biological molecules found in blood, other body fluids, or tissues that indicate a normal or abnormal condition, like CA 19-9 for pancreatic cancer.

Cholangiopancreatography (Endoscopic or Magnetic Resonance)
- Imaging techniques (ERCP or MRCP) used to diagnose conditions in the bile ducts, gallbladder, pancreas, and liver.

Cystic Neoplasms of the Pancreas
- Benign or malignant fluid-filled sacs in the pancreas, including intraductal papillary mucinous neoplasms (IPMNs).

Desmoplasia
- The growth of fibrous or connective tissue around a tumor, which can make pancreatic cancer more difficult to treat.

Endoscopic Ultrasound (EUS)
- A minimally invasive procedure that uses high-frequency sound waves to produce detailed images of the pancreas and obtain biopsy samples.

Enzyme Replacement Therapy
- The administration of pancreatic enzymes to aid digestion, often required for patients with pancreatic insufficiency.

FOLFIRINOX
- A chemotherapy regimen combining four drugs (5-FU, leucovorin, irinotecan, and oxaliplatin) used for advanced pancreatic cancer.

Gemcitabine
- A chemotherapy drug commonly used to treat pancreatic cancer.

Hypoglycemia
- Low blood sugar levels, which can occasionally occur in pancreatic neuroendocrine tumors (PNETs) that secrete insulin.

Islet Cells
- Hormone-producing cells in the pancreas; tumors in these cells are known as pancreatic neuroendocrine tumors (PNETs).

Jaundice
- Yellowing of the skin and eyes caused by elevated bilirubin levels, often linked to bile duct blockage by a pancreatic tumor.

KRAS Mutation
- A common genetic alteration in pancreatic cancer that promotes tumor growth.

Locally Advanced Pancreatic Cancer
- Cancer that has spread to nearby tissues or organs but has not metastasized to distant sites.

Neoadjuvant Therapy
- Treatment given before surgery to shrink tumors and increase the chances of a successful surgical resection.

Pancreaticoduodenectomy
- Another term for the Whipple procedure, a surgery to remove the head of the pancreas, part of the stomach, and nearby lymph nodes.

Proton Therapy
- A type of radiation therapy that uses protons instead of X-rays, which may reduce damage to surrounding healthy tissue.

Somatostatin Analogs
- Drugs like octreotide that can control symptoms and slow tumor growth in some pancreatic neuroendocrine tumors.

Targeted Therapy
- Cancer treatment designed to target specific molecules involved in tumor growth, such as PARP inhibitors for patients with BRCA mutations.

Venous Thromboembolism (VTE)
- Blood clots that form in the veins, a common complication in pancreatic cancer patients.

Zollinger-Ellison Syndrome
- A condition involving tumors (gastrinomas) in the pancreas or duodenum that cause excessive stomach acid production.

Hypercoagulability
- An increased tendency to form blood clots,

often seen in pancreatic cancer patients.

Lymphadenopathy

- Enlargement of lymph nodes, which may occur when cancer spreads to these structures.

Paraneoplastic Syndrome

- Symptoms that occur when cancer affects other parts of the body indirectly, such as changes in blood sugar levels or skin conditions.

Frequently Asked Questions (FAQ)

1. What are the early symptoms of pancreatic cancer?

Early symptoms can include abdominal pain, unexplained weight loss, jaundice (yellowing of the skin and eyes), changes in stool, and loss of appetite.

2. How is pancreatic cancer diagnosed?

Diagnosis typically involves imaging tests such as CT scans or MRIs, blood tests like CA 19-9 markers, and a biopsy to confirm the presence of cancer cells.

3. What are the treatment options for pancreatic cancer?

Treatment depends on the stage and may include surgery, chemotherapy, radiation therapy, targeted therapy, and immunotherapy. Palliative care is also an integral part of treatment at any stage.

4. Is pancreatic cancer hereditary?

While most cases are not hereditary, some individuals may have a genetic predisposition due to inherited mutations in genes like BRCA1, BRCA2, or others. Genetic testing can help assess risk.

5. What dietary changes are recommended for patients with pancreatic cancer?

A diet rich in easily digestible, nutrient-dense foods is recommended. Pancreatic enzyme supplements may be prescribed to aid digestion and absorption.

6. Are there clinical trials available for pancreatic cancer?

Yes, clinical trials are often available and may provide access to cutting-edge treatments. Patients should consult their healthcare team for guidance.

Resource Directory

Healthcare and Treatment:

American Cancer Society (ACS)
- Website: www.cancer.org
- Phone: 1-800-227-2345
- Services: Information on treatment options, support services, and research updates.

National Cancer Institute (NCI)
- Website: www.cancer.gov
- Phone: 1-800-422-6237 (1-800-4-CANCER)

- Services: Cancer resources, clinical trial information, and research publications.

Support Organizations

Pancreatic Cancer Action Network (PanCAN)
- Website: www.pancan.org
- Phone: 1-877-272-6226
- Address: 1500 Rosecrans Avenue, Suite 200, Manhattan Beach, CA 90266
- Services: Patient navigation, advocacy, research funding, and education.

Lustgarten Foundation
- Website: www.lustgarten.org
- Phone: 1-866-789-1000
- Address: 415 Crossways Park Drive, Suite D, Woodbury, NY 11797
- Services: Research funding and patient education.

CancerCare
- Website: www.cancercare.org
- Phone: 1-800-813-4673
- Address: 275 Seventh Avenue, New York, NY 10001
- Services: Free counseling, support groups, financial assistance, and workshops.

Online Communities

Inspire Pancreatic Cancer Community
- Website:www.inspire.com/groups/pancreatic-cancer-action-network
- Description: A forum for connecting with others affected by pancreatic cancer.

Cancer.net Community
- Website: www.cancer.net/support-and-social-media
- Description: Reliable resources and support network forums hosted by ASCO (American Society of Clinical Oncology).

Reddit: r/pancreaticcancer
- Website: www.reddit.com/r/pancreaticcancer
- Description: An informal platform for shared experiences and advice.

The appendices serve as a comprehensive resource for understanding pancreatic cancer and accessing the necessary tools for education, support, and advocacy. By utilizing these resources, individuals and families can make informed decisions and better navigate the complexities of this disease.

"Every day brings new hope, new strength, and new possibilities. You are stronger than you know, and your journey forward is one of courage and resilience."

Dear Reader,

Thank you for choosing my book! I hope you found it valuable and insightful. Reviews are a great way to help other readers discover this work and allow me to continue sharing more helpful content with you.

If you found this book useful, please consider leaving a positive review. Your feedback means so much to me and helps improve future publications.

Thank you for your support.

Warm regards,
Dr Mira Langford.